THE
EDGAR CAYCE WAY
OF OVERCOMING
MULTIPLE SCLEROSIS:
VIBRATORY MEDICINE

By
Dr. Dudley Delany

Foreword By
Dr. C. Norman Shealy

5th Ed (Rev)

THE
EDGAR CAYCE WAY
OF OVERCOMING
MULTIPLE SCLEROSIS:
VIBRATORY MEDICINE

By
Dr. Dudley Delany

Foreword By
Dr. C. Norman Shealy

5th Ed (Rev)

Published by:
A Division of
Amazon.com

Publisher's Cataloging in Publication Data:

Delany, Dudley, 1940-

The Edgar Cayce Way of Overcoming Multiple Sclerosis: Vibratory Medicine/by Dr. Dudley Delany, 5th edition (revised)
Library of Congress Catalog Card
Number: 99-70273
120 p.: ill.; 22 cm.
Includes appendix, bibliography, and
index; paperback ($14.95); illustrated
ISBN 10-1495294722 13-9781495294723

1. Multiple sclerosis–Popular works.
2. Multiple sclerosis–Alternative treatment.
3. Cayce, Edgar, 1877-1945.
4. Delany, Dudley.
I. Title.
RC377.D45 1999   616.83406

DEDICATION

This book is affectionately dedicated to the patients and staff on the spinal cord injury ward of the V.A. Medical Center in Hampton, Virginia, where the author ministered for seven years in the nursing service.

ACKNOWLEDGMENTS

Special thanks go to Virginia Smith and her daughter D.D. for their extraordinary encouragement and support in producing this volume.

IMPORTANT NOTE TO READERS WITH MS

It is essential that the treatment recommendations contained in this publication be implemented with the knowledge, consent, and cooperation of your attending physician, so that he or she can propose any appropriate modifications, closely monitor your progress, adjust your medication schedule if necessary, intervene as needed with helpful advice and suggestions, and document whatever results may be obtained. In addition, it is possible that your experience with vibratory medicine may inspire him or her to undertake *desperately* needed research in a field that has the potential of bringing health, help, and healing to *millions*. For vibratory medicine has been found to be effective in treating not only multiple sclerosis, but many other conditions as well, some of which (such as muscular dystrophy and Lou Gehrig's disease) are, on the whole, even more serious and debilitating than MS.

FOREWORD

Like Dr. Delany, I have been a student of Edgar Cayce for many years. Much of the health advice that Cayce gave has been shown to be effective in a variety of situations. This book is, however, to my knowledge, the first documentation of continuing benefit from the very simple and safe treatments Cayce proposed well over 70 years ago.

Modern conventional medicine has relatively little to offer individuals with MS. Those medications currently in use to treat it carry a number of undesirable "side effects" or complications, and certainly are not curative.

If I had MS, I hope that I would have the wisdom, no matter what else I might do, to incorporate the Cayce suggestions.

The extensive comments about good nutrition in MS are themselves worthy of considerable study.

You have nothing to lose following the program that Dr. Delany has outlined from the Cayce material, but you potentially have everything to gain. Indeed, there is a great deal to celebrate and a lot to recommend in following the advice in this book.

C. Norman Shealy, M.D., Ph.D.
Founder, The American
Holistic Medical Association

PREFACE

Based on the work of the late Edgar Cayce, *vibratory medicine is a very mild form of electrotherapy which treats human ills by administering – in a painless and non-invasive manner – the essential essence or "vibration" of certain substances having medicinal properties.* It is a way of administering substances which are relatively *toxic* to the body (like *gold* in the treatment of rheumatoid arthritis) *without* adverse effects; it is a way of administering substances in which the body may be *deficient* (like *iron* in the treatment of anemia) *without* using food supplements; it is a way of administering substances to which the body may be *allergic* (like *iodine* in the treatment of goiter) *without* causing allergic reactions. It represents a totally new idea, a totally new concept, a totally new approach to administering selected medicinal agents, and it has the potential of *revolutionizing* medicine.

At least two devices currently exist to accomplish the goals of vibratory medicine, the "radial appliance" and the "wet cell battery."

These pages relate the manner in which I and others used vibratory medicine to overcome *multiple sclerosis*, a chronic, sometimes disabling neurological disorder of unknown cause that afflicts an estimated 350,000 to 500,000 Americans.

It is hoped that this publication will be a blessing, a comfort, and an encouragement to those who seek an "alternative approach" to defeating this disturbing, sometimes devastating disease for which, at the present time, medical science has no cure.

Dudley Delany, R.N., M.A., D.C.
Muncy, Pennsylvania

TABLE OF CONTENTS

CHAPTER 1

THE EDGAR CAYCE LEGACY

Edgar Cayce was born near Hopkinsville, Kentucky, in 1877. A man of humble means and with very little formal education, he became a photographer, married a delicate, sensitive woman, and eventually fathered three boys. A devout Christian, he became a Sunday School teacher, and read the Bible through once for every year of his life. His hobbies included fishing, bowling, golf, and playing cards.

What really set Edgar Cayce apart from the mass of humanity was the fact that, at the age of thirteen, he encountered an angel who asked him what he *most* wanted in life. The young man replied that he wanted to help people, especially children. At the age of twenty-one, Edgar Cayce developed the astonishing ability to enter a self-induced hypnotic trance in which he could *diagnose illnesses* and *prescribe treatments* which, though usually unorthodox, were often amazingly effective.

These trance discourses came to be known as "readings," and they proved to be so helpful to so many that it was decided early on to record, preserve, and study them.

When Edgar Cayce died in 1945, he left a legacy of over 14,000 readings, all of which are on file (and also on CD-ROM computer disc) at the Association for Research and Enlightenment, 215 67th Street, Virginia Beach, VA 23451. The A.R.E. makes available to any interested party not only the readings, but also the many books, articles, audio cassettes, and video presentations based on them. It also publishes a quarterly magazine.

While some of the readings deal with dream analysis, Bible interpretation, future events and other subjects, the majority address most of the ills to which flesh is heir.

Included in those ills were numerous health problems for which the readings recommended the "vibratory" administration of various substances using either the radial appliance or the wet cell battery. The design, construction, operation, maintenance, care, and use of these devices is based solely on information provided by the readings.

Unlike the light bulb and the phonograph, the appliances were not "invented." Rather, they were *given* – as a gift of *grace* to the world – through a sleeping photographer – by some "source" that apparently has great wisdom, great compassion, and great love for a suffering and afflicted humanity.

For a fascinating account of Edgar Cayce's remarkable life, work, and ministry, read *The Edgar Cayce Story – There is a River* by Thomas Sugrue (obtainable by calling 1-800-723-1112). You can use that number to purchase numerous outstanding Cayce-related books and videos.

They that wait upon the LORD shall renew their strength; they shall mount up with wings as eagles; they shall run and not be weary; and they shall walk, and not faint.

Isaiah 40:31

CHAPTER 2

THE RADIAL
APPLIANCE

INTRODUCTION

The radial appliance (also referred to as the impedance device, the radio-active appliance, and the dry cell) was recommended in over 900 readings in the treatment of such conditions as nervous tension, poor circulation, insomnia, vaginitis, neurasthenia, debilitation, hypertension, migraine headaches, psoriasis, deafness, obesity, tic douloureux, tuberculosis, leukemia, and sterility.

CONSTRUCTION DETAILS

Although minor variations exist between models of different manufacturers, in general, the appliance consists of a metal container (2" X 2-1/4" X 6-1/2") containing two high-carbon-content rectangular steel rods (each 1/4" X 1/2" X 5") separated by two pieces of glass (each 1/16" X 1/2" X 5") and surrounded on four sides by four pieces of carbon (two are 1/4" X 1/2" X 5" and two are 1/4" X 1-3/16" X 5"). This carbon-steel-glass "sandwich" is wrapped like a cocoon in tape and immersed in charcoal particles. Each steel rod attaches to a terminal on the outside of the appliance.

The appliance also comes equipped with a round, slightly concave copper electrode (1" in diameter), a round, slightly concave nickel electrode (2-1/2" in diameter), a four-ounce-capacity "solution jar" containing a loop (3/16" in diameter) made of hollow lead tubing in the shape of a "U" (other shapes are also available but are more fragile and harder to clean), and appropriate connecting wire (see Figure 1).

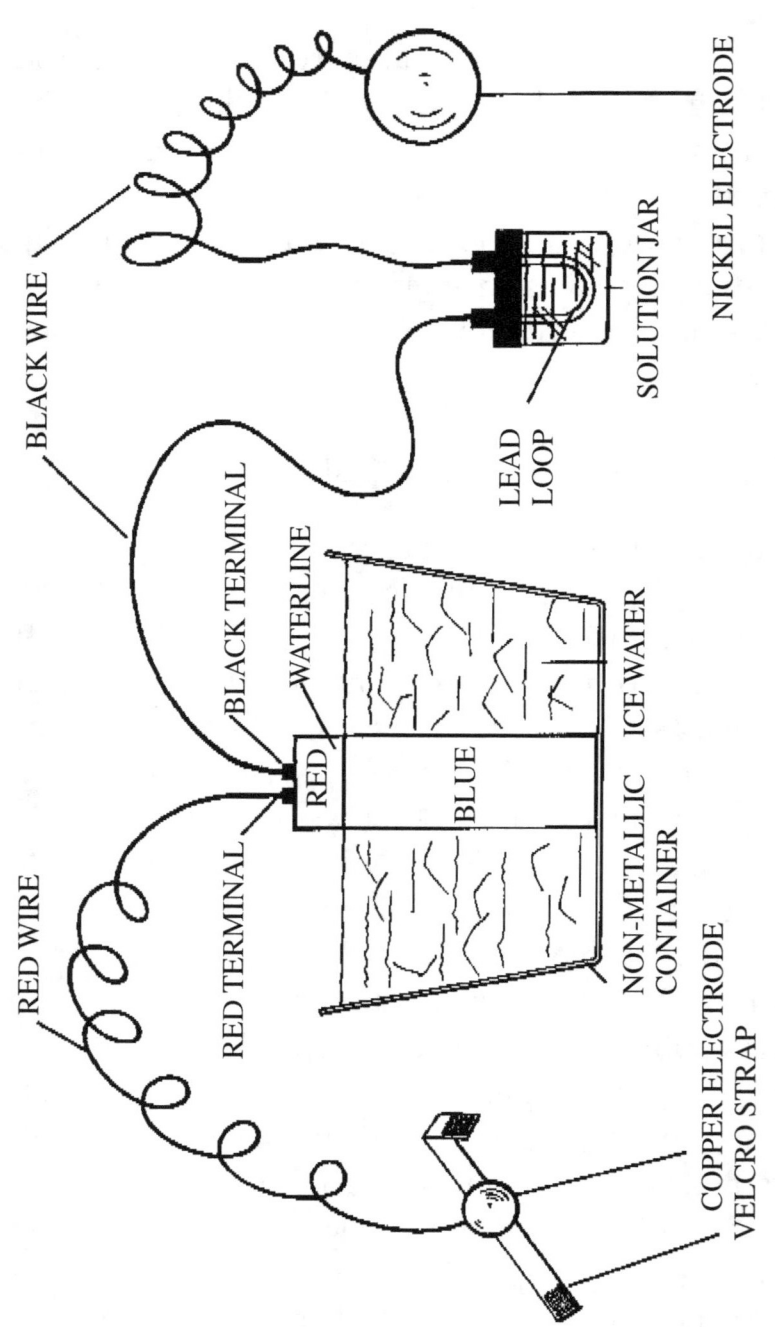

FIGURE 1: RADIAL APPLIANCE WITH SOLUTION JAR.

BLACK WIRE

BLACK TERMINAL

WATERLINE

RED WIRE

RED TERMINAL

RED

BLUE

NON-METALLIC
CONTAINER

ICE WATER

LEAD
LOOP

SOLUTION JAR

NICKEL ELECTRODE

COPPER ELECTRODE

VELCRO STRAP

HOW THE RADIAL APPLIANCE IS USED

There are two ways in which the radial appliance may be utilized, *without* the solution jar and *with* the solution jar.

Use of the appliance *without* the solution jar is intended mainly to promote relaxation, improve circulation, and balance the body mentally, physically, and spiritually. For a discussion of how the appliance is connected to the body and utilized in this way, the interested reader is referred to literature available from the parties listed in the Appendix.

Use of the appliance *with* the solution jar is intended mainly to introduce into the body the essential essence or vibration of some particular substance (such as iodine, silver, iron, quinine, or gold) *without* introducing the actual substance itself. One might liken it to introducing the scent of a rose but not the rose itself, or the music of a violin but not the violin itself, or the warmth and glow of a lighted candle but not the candle itself. This task is accomplished (as can be seen in Figure 1) by routing the flow of energy from the *black* (normally negative) terminal on the appliance *through the solution jar*, where the vibration of the desired substance is acquired. Leaving the solution jar, the energy is then deposited on the nickel electrode (which is often placed on the abdomen near the navel). It then enters and flows through the body, is collected by the copper electrode (which is often attached to the wrist or ankle), and returned to the appliance via the *red* (normally positive) terminal.

Although a "subtle" energy component may also be involved, the nature of this energy is a naturally occurring form of electricity produced by the body itself. The appliance merely induces and modulates its flow.

The substance to be placed in the solution jar varies depending on the condition to be treated. The one most frequently recommended, however, was *gold* (in the form of a dilute solution of gold chloride). The readings stated that the vibratory administration of gold would help rejuvenate *any* organ that was "delinquent" in its action. How that occurs, and what connection gold has with tissue growth, repair, healing, and regeneration is not clear.

STEPS IN OPERATING THE APPLIANCE

In setting up and using the radial appliance,

(1) pour the solution you wish to use into the solution jar and cover it with the *bare* lid;

(2) change the solution in the jar after *fifteen* uses;

(3) keep the solution jar covered with the bare lid and in a *dark* place when not in use;

(4) never allow the solution jar to come into direct contact with sunlight;

(5) before use, carefully sand and polish the loop and the rim and cup of both electrodes with 600 grit sandpaper (giving them a final wipe with tissue paper);

(6) always use a protective (dust) mask when sanding (available at most hardware stores and pharmacies);

(7) before use, place the appliance into a suitable non-metallic container (such as a plastic paint pail); fill the container with *ice* to the waterline on the appliance; then fill the container with *water* to the waterline;

(8) never allow water to come up over the top of the appliance or to cover the attached wiring;

(9) allow the appliance to cool down in the ice water *twenty minutes* before attachment to the body;

(10) *five minutes* before attaching the appliance to the body, put the loop into the solution jar and screw down the lid; connect the solution jar to the *black terminal* on the appliance; then connect the nickel electrode to the solution jar;

(11) begin your session on the appliance by assuming a relaxed, comfortable supine or, preferably, prone position in a location free from distractions or disturbances; connect the copper electrode to the

red terminal on the appliance; then apply the copper electrode to the body;

(12) if applying the copper electrode to an extremity, use the Velcro strap to hold it in place (make the strap loose enough so as not to impede circulation);

(13) if applying the copper electrode elsewhere, secure it with adhesive tape or other suitable means;

(14) after the copper electrode has been properly situated, wait a couple of minutes and then apply the nickel electrode, securing it with adhesive tape or other expedient;

(15) always be sure to apply the copper electrode *first*;

(16) insure that both electrodes lie *flat* against the skin;

(17) maintain each session for a period of *thirty minutes*;

(18) occupy your time on the appliance in prayer, meditation, and/or reading the Bible or other inspirational literature;

(19) when your session is over, remove the nickel and then the copper electrode from the body; disconnect the electrodes from the appliance; disconnect the black wiring from the solution jar; dry off the loop and carefully sand and polish it

with 600 grit sandpaper (giving it a final wipe with tissue paper); remove the appliance from the ice water, dry it off, and place it in the sun; then carefully sand and polish the rim and cup of both electrodes with 600 grit sandpaper (giving them a final wipe with tissue paper);

(20) protect the appliance from the elements if placed in the sun *outdoors*;

(21) never allow the electrodes and their associated wiring to touch, whether attached to the appliance or not;

(22) never allow the appliance to come into contact with anything metallic;

(23) if attempting to administer more than one substance vibratorially, for each solution, provide a separate jar, loop, and nickel electrode; and

(24) patiently and persistently persevere in the use of the appliance.

CHAPTER 3

THE WET CELL BATTERY

INTRODUCTION

The wet cell battery (also known as the wet cell appliance) was recommended in about 975 readings in the treatment of such conditions as Down's syndrome, spinal cord injuries, scleroderma, stroke, alcoholism, major depression, schizophrenia, color blindness, Parkinson's disease, muscular dystrophy, Lou Gehrig's disease, Alzheimer's disease, rheumatoid arthritis, cancer, polio, and multiple sclerosis.

CONSTRUCTION DETAILS

There are currently two types of wet cell batteries on the market, one with short (8" to 10") poles, and one with long (14" to 16") poles. The short-pole version is illustrated in Figure 1. The long-pole version is similar in design and operation, but is taller and more slender in appearance.

What we have in Figure 1 is essentially the configuration of a simple wet cell battery, consisting of two cylindrical rods or "poles," each measuring 1/2" in diameter and between 8" and 10" long, one made of copper and the other of nickel, suspended in an electrolytic solution. The container holds two gallons and has a matching lid (both are made of non-metallic material).

On top of each pole is a terminal. The one attached to the copper pole is *red* and represents the *positive* side of the battery. The one attached to the nickel pole is *black* and represents the *negative* side.

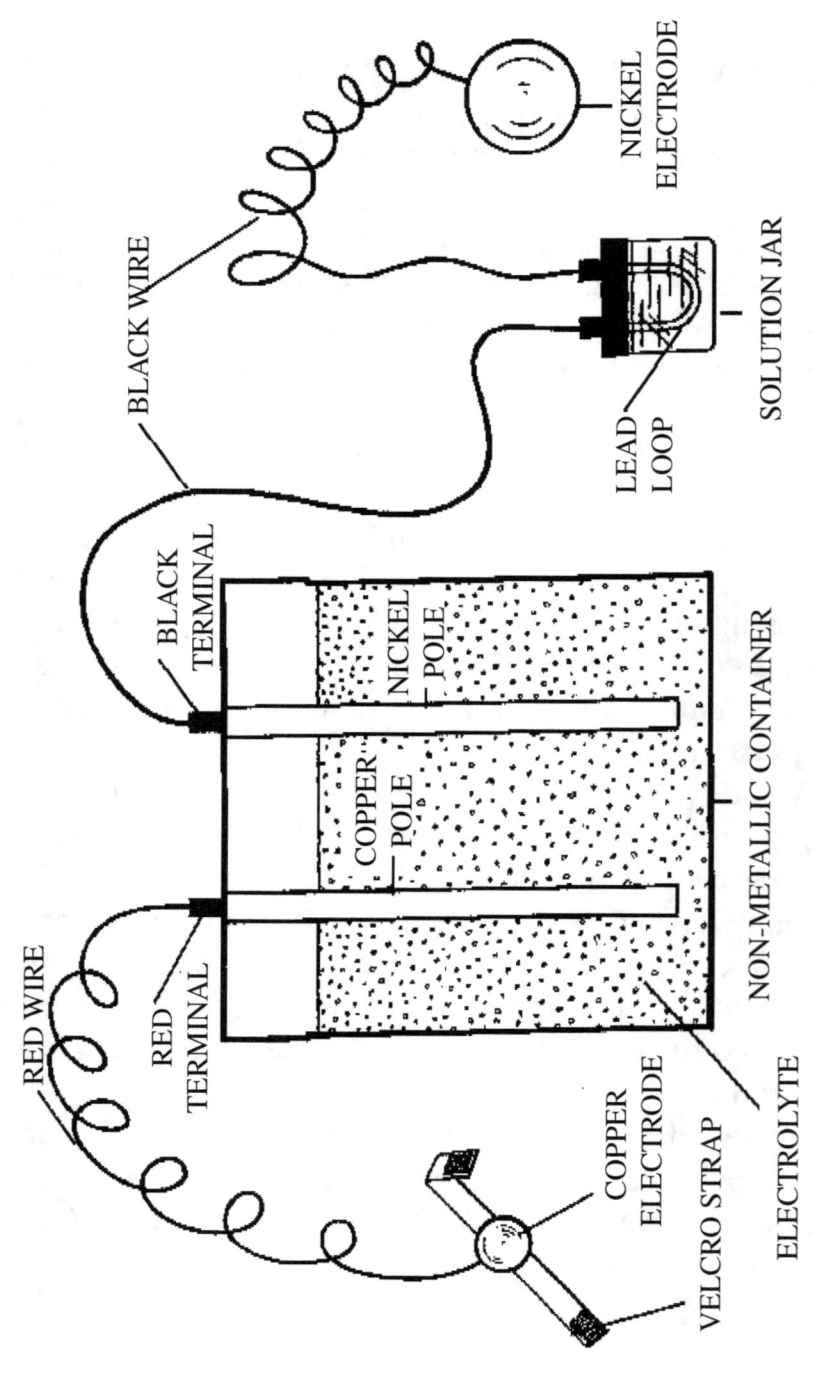

FIGURE 1: WET CELL BATTERY (SHORT-POLE TYPE)

The wet cell battery comes equipped with a round, slightly concave copper electrode (1" in diameter), a round, slightly concave nickel electrode (2-1/2" in diameter), a four-ounce-capacity solution jar containing a loop made of hollow lead tubing (3/16" in diameter) in the shape of a "U" (other shapes are also available but are more fragile and harder to clean), and appropriate connecting wire.

ELECTROLYTE PREPARATION

Place the container on some newspaper outdoors or under an exhaust fan. Wearing vinyl gloves, pour 1-1/2 gallons of distilled water into the container. Then slowly add (stirring constantly with a wooden stick or utensil) the following ingredients in the order named:

(1)   1-1/2 pounds of copper sulfate,
(2)   4 ounces of sulfuric acid (25% solution), and
(3)   5.3 grams of zinc particles.

When all the copper sulfate has dissolved, *slowly* add 1/2 pound of willow charcoal, stirring constantly until it is completely dispersed into the solution. Then put the poles into the electrolyte and the lid on the container.

The exact amount of zinc necessary in the electrolyte frequently varied from person to person and from condition to condition. The figure shown above and those given in Chapter 4 are based on certain *MS readings* which specify that a "regular" charge requires 3 drams (5.3 grams), and that a "double strength" charge requires 6 drams (10.6 grams) of zinc.

HOW THE WET CELL BATTERY IS USED

The wet cell battery is usually utilized *with* the solution jar. Its primary function, therefore, is the vibratory administration of various medicinal agents.

As can be seen in Figure 1, energy flows from the *black* (negative) terminal on the appliance *through the solution jar*, where the vibration of the desired substance is acquired. It is then deposited on the nickel electrode (which is often placed on the abdomen near the navel), flows through the body, is collected by the copper electrode (which is often placed on a particular spinal vertebra), and returned to the appliance via the *red* (positive) terminal.

The nature of this energy is frankly electrical (although a subtle energy component may also be involved) and it can easily be measured with the appropriate instruments (*do not* measure the voltage output just prior to using the device, however). Typically, the wet cell battery develops between 20 and 35 millivolts of electrical potential.

In comparison to the radial appliance, there is very little mystery surrounding the wet cell battery – everything is out in the open; we learn about batteries in school; and we use them to start our cars, power our flashlights, etc. In addition, the readings indicated that the wet cell, by its very nature, actually contributes useful, *neuroavailable* energy to the body (over and above the vibration of various substances), whereas the radial appliance does not.

STEPS IN OPERATING THE WET CELL

In setting up and using the wet cell battery,

(1) after electrolyte preparation, place the appliance where it need not be moved to utilize it, such as on a nightstand next to and about halfway between the foot and head of your bed (let it stand for 24 hours before use);

(2) keep the appliance from direct exposure to sunlight if it is made of clear plastic or glass;

(3) pour the solution you wish to use into the solution jar and cover it with the *bare* lid;

(4) change the solution in the solution jar after *fifteen* uses;

(5) keep the solution jar covered with the bare lid and in a *dark* place when not in use;

(6) never allow the solution jar to come into direct contact with sunlight;

(7) before use, carefully sand and polish the loop and the rim and cup of both electrodes with 600 grit sandpaper (giving them a final wipe with tissue paper);

(8) always use a protective (dust) mask when sanding (and also when doing dusty housework);

(9) *twenty minutes* before the attachment of the wet cell to the body, put the loop into the solution

jar and screw down the lid; connect the solution jar to the *black terminal* on the appliance; connect the nickel electrode to the solution jar; then connect the copper electrode to the *red terminal* on the appliance;

(10) begin your session on the wet cell by assuming a relaxed, comfortable supine or, preferably, prone position in a location free from distractions or disturbances; then apply the copper electrode to the body;

(11) if applying the copper electrode to an extremity, use the Velcro strap to hold it in place (make the strap loose enough so as not to impede circulation);

(12) if applying the copper electrode elsewhere, secure it with adhesive tape or other suitable means;

(13) after the copper electrode has been properly situated, apply the nickel electrode, securing it with adhesive tape or other expedient;

(14) always be sure to apply the copper electrode *first*;

(15) insure that both electrodes lie *flat* against the skin;

(16) maintain each session for a period of *thirty minutes*;

(17) occupy your time on the wet cell in prayer, meditation, and/or reading the Bible or other inspirational literature;

(18) when your session is over, remove the nickel and then the copper electrode from the body; disconnect the electrodes from the appliance; disconnect the black wiring from the solution jar; dry off the loop, and carefully sand and polish it with 600 grit sandpaper (giving it a final wipe with tissue paper); then carefully sand and polish the rim and cup of both electrodes with 600 grit sandpaper (giving them a final wipe with tissue paper);

(19) place the loop, wiring, and electrodes in the sun between sessions (protect them from the elements if placed *outdoors*);

(20) never allow the poles or the electrodes and their associated wiring to touch, whether attached to the appliance or not;

(21) after *thirty* uses, discard the electrolyte; clean out and dry the container; remove all accumulations from the poles with 120 grit sandpaper, a wire brush, and, if necessary, a file (giving them a final wipe with tissue paper); then prepare the electrolyte for the next series of treatments;

(22) if attempting to administer more than one substance vibratorially, for each solution, provide a separate jar, loop, and nickel electrode; and

(23) patiently and persistently persevere in the use of the appliance.

CHAPTER 4

WHAT THE READINGS
SAY ABOUT
MULTIPLE SCLEROSIS

INTRODUCTION

Edgar Cayce gave scores of readings for dozens of persons who appeared to be suffering from multiple sclerosis. He also gave one reading (907-1) for a physician who sought specific information on its cause and treatment. Most of these readings are reproduced in the seven volume set of A.R.E. Circulating Files on MS (any or all of which may be borrowed or purchased by calling 1-800-333-4499).

THE CAUSE AND TREATMENT
OF MULTIPLE SCLEROSIS

The readings recognized many types of MS, but cited the usual cause as *a deficiency of gold in the body.*

In what is apparently the most common scenario, a glandular disturbance creates a hormonal deficit in the bloodstream which prevents the *liver* (in association with the spleen and pancreas) from properly assimilating the trace amounts of gold normally present in the diet. Without sufficient quantities of gold in the system, certain neurotrophic glands (possibly unicellular) located in various segments of the spine – including the sacrum and coccyx (tail bone) – become incapable of secreting that which is necessary to maintain the structural and functional integrity of nerve cells. The result is a neurodestructive process that begins in the lower portion of the spinal cord and gradually progresses upward to the brain. In males, the lack of gold also hinders the normal production of sperm cells, causing a measure of sterility. This whole sequence of events is based on a congenital predisposition, and may be precipitated by trauma (particularly to the spine), vertebral subluxations, liver

28

problems, local or systemic infections, negative attitudes and/or emotions, environmental toxins, ingesting calcium chloride (a common preservative), childbearing, and other significant stressors. The congenital predisposition may be due to heredity, adverse conditions surrounding conception, or both.

In another scenario, the gold deficiency stems from *inadequate dietary intake* of that mineral (due, for example, to poor eating habits, fad diets, fasting, and ingesting nutritionally deficient food).

Still another scenario involves gold deficiency related to *malabsorptive conditions* (such as celiac disease, discussed on pages 71-73).

A *combination* of these and other scenarios (especially those involving iron, silver, and fat) is also possible.

To correct the gold deficiency, the readings usually recommended instilling gold into the body vibratorially via the wet cell. The body responds to gold in its vibratory state by increasing assimilation of that and perhaps other nutrients. Massage therapy (aimed primarily at stimulating and energizing nerves) and close attention to diet were also frequently recommended.

TREATING MULTIPLE SCLEROSIS WITH THE WET CELL BATTERY

The specifics of using the wet cell battery in the treatment of MS generally varied somewhat from case to case, but one effective approach might be to

(1)   employ the device in continuous 30-day cycles;
(2)   use a three ounce solution of gold chloride (available from the suppliers listed in the Appendix)

29

in the solution jar (in a concentration of one grain of gold chloride per ounce of distilled water);

(3) apply the copper electrode alternately to the *ninth dorsal* vertebra one day, and to the *fourth lumbar* vertebra the next day; and

(4) always place the nickel electrode on the abdomen slightly above and to the right of the navel (as illustrated on page 49).

HINTS ON PLACING THE COPPER ELECTRODE

In addition to the sacrum and coccyx, the vertebral column consists of seven cervical (neck) vertebrae, twelve dorsal (thoracic) vertebrae, and five lumbar (low back) vertebrae.

The row of "bumps" you see running up and down the middle of a person's back are the *spinous processes* (rearmost projections) of the vertebrae.

To locate the *fourth lumbar* vertebra, draw an imaginary line across the small of the back between the tops of the iliac crests. It should intersect the vertebral column at about the level of the fourth lumbar vertebra. The spinous process of this vertebra is the alternate site for placing the copper electrode.

The largest projection at the base of the back of the neck is usually the spinous process of the seventh cervical vertebra. Just below it is the spinous process of the first dorsal vertebra.

To locate the *ninth dorsal* vertebra, one method is to count down nine bumps from the first dorsal vertebra. Depending on the physique of the person with whom you are working, however, that method may be difficult or impossible. An alternate method is to have the person sit erect. Draw an imaginary line between the lower tips of the scapulae (shoulder blades). It should intersect the vertebral column at about the level of the seventh dorsal vertebra. Count down two bumps and you should be at the level of ninth dorsal vertebra. The copper electrode should be placed initially on the spinous process of this vertebra.

MASSAGE IN THE TREATMENT
OF MULTIPLE SCLEROSIS

After each session on the wet cell battery, it is suggested that massage therapy be administered (preferably on a massage table by someone close to you) as follows:

(1)   as a lubricant, use Aura Glow or a comparable mixture of oils (available from suppliers listed in the Appendix);
(2)   gently but thoroughly massage the oil (as much as the body will absorb) into the skin beginning at the base of the skull and working down the neck and back on both sides of the spine, across the lumbar and sacral areas, into the gluteal muscles, and down both legs to the feet and toes;
(3)   massage the shoulders, arms, and hands;
(4)   use mostly a circular or rotary motion;
(5)   keep a positive attitude that *good is being accomplished*; and
(6)   maintain each session for a period of thirty minutes.

DIET IN THE TREATMENT
OF MULTIPLE SCLEROSIS

Proper diet is critical in the treatment of MS. To that end, it is recommended that you

(1) avoid alcoholic beverages;
(2) avoid ingesting any products containing caffeine or genetically modified ingredients (watch this video: http://tinyurl.com/dump-gmos);
(3) avoid ingesting anything containing white sugar (as a substitute, the readings suggest using beet sugar, saccharin, or raw honey);
(4) avoid smoked foods;
(5) avoid foods containing nitrates, nitrites, benzoate of soda, calcium chloride, MSG, and other chemical additives and preservatives;
(6) avoid fried food (http://tinyurl.com/dump-fries);
(7) never eat pork;
(8) never drink carbonated beverages;
(9) do not eat beef (unless 100% grass-fed organic);
(10) eat seafood and shellfish often (also good occasionally are liver, and poultry with the skin removed);
(11) avoid white rice and potatoes;
(12) fresh raw fruits, vegetables, and their juices should be part of your daily diet (for lunch, I might have a can of carrot juice);
(13) avoid spicy foods;
(14) avoid gluten (read pgs 71-73 and watch this video: http://tinyurl.com/dump-gluten);
(15) eat quantities of lettuce every day (it acts as a blood purifier);
(16) do not combine whole grain cereals or dairy products with citrus fruit or citrus fruit juices at the same meal;

(17) salads (preferably mixed with unflavored gelatin) made with grated or chopped *raw* carrots, lettuce, celery, watercress, radishes, onions, vine ripened or canned tomatoes, and *cooked* beets are excellent (I may have a large one for dinner with an extra virgin olive oil/herb seasoned dressing);

(18) avoid products containing saturated fat, such as butter, lard, whole milk, and cheese (skim milk and nonfat yogurt are alright, provided you are not lactose intolerant or allergic to dairy products);

(19) in regard to eggs, eat only the *yolks*, and make sure they are thoroughly cooked (for breakfast, I might have a hard-boiled, jumbo egg yolk sprinkled with unflavored gelatin, sunflower seeds, and bee pollen on toasted brown rice bread with lettuce and applesauce);

(20) do not eat if you are excited, angry, upset, or excessively fatigued;

(21) take a liver extract capsule with each meal (call Swanson Vitamins at 1-800-437-4248);

(22) never ingest anything prepared or stored in aluminum;

(23) eat a few almonds every day;

(24) use little or no salt;

(25) avoid *raw* apples unless you are on the apple cleansing diet (see Question 8 on page 70);

(26) take, half an hour before breakfast, in continuous cycles of five days on and five days off, one drop of Atomidine (available from suppliers listed in the Appendix) in half a glass of water;

(27) take a really good multivitamin/mineral supplement (or its equivalent) daily;

(28) avoid candy, cake, pies, pastries, and ice cream;

(29) try to drink six to eight glasses of water daily;

(30) avoid products containing vinegar (such as pickles, relish, ketchup, mayonnaise, and salad dressing);

(31) have some unflavored gelatin with every meal (it aids absorption of nutrients);

(32) do not cook with condiments, including salt (it destroys much of the vitamin content of food);

(33) drink half a glass of warm water upon arising in the morning (it helps rid the body of toxins);

(34) because digestion begins in the mouth, chew your food thoroughly (even liquids should be chewed two or three times before swallowing);

(35) take a digestive enzymes capsule with every meal;

(36) avoid high fructose corn syrup;

(37) do not eat bananas unless vine ripened in your vicinity;

(38) have at least one leafy vegetable to every one of the pod variety;

(39) avoid any vegetable oil that has been hydrogenated (e.g., vegetable shortening and margarine) or otherwise processed or refined (with the exception of palm oil and coconut oil, which are both high in saturated fat, "cold pressed" oils are alright, and extra virgin olive oil is especially recommended);

(40) insofar as possible, eat mostly raw, organic, locally grown foods; and

(41) for more Cayce dietary information, read *Nourishing the Body Temple* by Simone Gabbay, R.N.C.P. (see http://tinyurl.com/nourishing-the-body).

The preceding recommendations represent Plan "A" in the treatment of MS and pertain to *mild* cases in which there is no appreciable paralysis or disability – "just" the annoying signs and symptoms of the type listed on page 46.

TREATING CASES OF MODERATE SEVERITY (PLAN "B")

In treating cases of *moderate* severity (characterized by a significant degree of paralysis and disability but without total loss of the ability to ambulate), it is suggested that you adhere to Plan "A" with the following exceptions:

(1) increase the duration of the massage therapy session to forty minutes; and
(2) use the following ingredients in the wet cell battery:

> (A) 2 pounds of copper sulfate,
> (B) 4 ounces of sulfuric acid (33.33% solution),
> (C) 7.1 grams of zinc particles, and
> (D) 1/2 pound of willow charcoal.

TREATING SEVERE CASES (PLAN "C")

In treating *severe* cases of MS (characterized by extensive paralysis and disability with no ability to ambulate), it is suggested that you adhere to Plan "A" with the following exceptions:

(1) increase the duration of the massage therapy sessions to fifty minutes; and
(2) use the following ingredients in the wet cell battery:

> (A) 2-1/2 pounds of copper sulfate,

(B) 4 ounces of sulfuric acid (41.75% solution),
(C) 8.8 grams of zinc particles, and
(D) 1/2 pound of willow charcoal.

DURATION OF TREATMENT

Treating multiple sclerosis using the Cayce approach is typically a long-term proposition. Depending on the severity of the condition, it could take up to seven years (or more) to achieve the maximum therapeutic effect (although definite signs of improvement should occur within the first several months).

WHAT I DID

In regard to the preceding treatment recommendations, I received massage therapy only sporadically (due to the expense and inconvenience involved), was sometimes remiss in following the proper diet (due to a lack of self-control), chose the radial appliance as the vehicle for administering gold vibratorially (for reasons discussed in Chapter 5), and took a different approach to placing the copper electrode (for reasons discussed in Chapter 6).

CHAPTER 5

THE RELATIVE MERITS
OF EACH APPLIANCE

THE WET CELL BATTERY

From all indications, the wet cell battery is clearly the "fast track" in terms of treating multiple sclerosis. It is the device recommended by the readings; it is the more powerful instrument; it does not depend on the body for its source of energy; it instills useful energy into the body; and it is probably less sensitive to negative thoughts and emotions on the part of the person using it. It is undoubtedly the treatment of choice in most cases of multiple sclerosis.

THE RADIAL APPLIANCE

If you have a relatively mild, nonparalytic form of multiple sclerosis, you *might* – as I did – "get by" with the radial appliance. It can be very effective as a weapon in the arsenal of vibratory medicine, particularly if the person using it has chosen a "spiritual path" and is in general accord with its use. It is considerably less expensive to operate, especially on a long-term basis; it is portable; there are no chemicals to mix periodically; when and if you finish using it to treat your MS, you can use it to your advantage *without* the solution jar; and you can even alternate its use both with and without the solution jar.

In my own case, I had consistently utilized the radial appliance for many years *without* the solution jar. Therefore, I was thoroughly familiar with its operation;

my body was accustomed to the device; and I felt quite comfortable using it.

It was for the above reasons that I initially chose the radial appliance to treat my multiple sclerosis.

In retrospect, I believe that the wet cell battery would have produced more positive results more quickly, and, from that standpoint, would have been the wiser choice.

For persons at risk for developing MS (such as those with close relatives with the disease), the radial appliance might be an appropriate choice for use *prophylactically* (along the lines suggested in Chapter 7).

The radial appliance might also be a more appropriate choice in treating *children* and certain unusually *sensitive individuals* (who might find the wet cell battery too "harsh").

Finally, the radial appliance would make a good substitute for the wet cell when you are *traveling*.

Trust in the LORD with all thine heart; and lean not unto thine own understanding. In all thy ways acknowledge him, and he shall direct thy paths.

Proverbs 3:5-6

CHAPTER 6

A WORD ABOUT
ELECTRODE PLACEMENT

INTRODUCTION

In the practice of vibratory medicine, there are two main approaches to attaching the electrodes of either appliance to the body, the *general* and the *specific*.

THE GENERAL APPROACH

Regardless of which device you are using, if the nickel electrode is placed near the navel, and the copper electrode rotates around the extremities (as exemplified in Chapter 7), you are using the *general* approach.

This technique is particularly effective in the treatment of *widespread* conditions, such as systemic infections, and in the simultaneous treatment of *more than one* condition, such as multiple sclerosis and a heart problem.

This approach will probably *always* work to help alleviate *any* condition amenable to vibratory medicine. However, depending on the nature of the condition, it may take longer and be less effective than the specific approach.

In this technique, attachment of the copper electrode to the body is relatively easy to make, especially if – as in my case – you happen to be working *alone*.

It was for the above reasons that I chose the general approach in my use of the radial appliance.

THE SPECIFIC APPROACH

This technique encompasses virtually all other variations of electrode placement.

Here, the attempt is made to focus *specifically* on a particular organ or system that is malfunctioning.

For example, in treating MS with the wet cell battery (as discussed in Chapter 4), you will notice that the electrodes are always placed in such a way that healthful energies *must* flow through important nerve centers.

As another example, in treating certain female problems, the readings recommend placing the nickel electrode over the pubic area, and the copper electrode over the fourth lumbar vertebra. Here again, healthful energies *must* bathe the affected organs.

This approach, however, usually works best in treating one problem at a time, and you may need the assistance of another person to *properly* place the copper electrode.

Seek ye the LORD while he may be found, call ye upon him while he is near.

Isaiah 55:6

CHAPTER 7

HOW I OVERCAME MS USING THE RADIAL APPLIANCE

INTRODUCTION

During the summer of 1991, I began to notice an occasional numbness in some of my fingers.

Unexplained muscle spasms and tremors also began to occur.

Once, I felt what seemed to be a powerful electric shock go down my spine (Lhermitte's sign).

At times, I would be walking along on a smooth, flat surface and, for no apparent reason, stumble.

Occasionally, I would chew a bite of food, attempt to swallow it, and *nothing* would happen.

I was beginning to choke on fluids that "went down the wrong pipe."

My speech was becoming a little slurred.

Once in a while, my face would contort in an embarrassing and uncontrollable manner.

I was having trouble completely emptying my bladder.

Sometimes, I would experience episodes of blurred vision, see flashes of light, and have an unscratchable itch behind my eyes.

My memory was beginning to fail.

I would often be unreasonably fatigued, inordinately depressed, and, on a few occasions, euphoric without cause.

During minor confrontations with co-workers, I tended to become almost hysterical.

My symptoms were aggravated by hot showers, heating pads and hot water bottles, hot environments, stress, certain viral infections, and, in particular, by a flu shot I received in the late fall of 1991.

It was obvious that I was developing a very serious and pervasive health problem.

It was *multiple sclerosis*.

THE REGIMEN THAT WORKED FOR ME

Based on my study of the Cayce readings, I decided to employ the radial appliance (beginning in November of 1991) in continuous cycles of 28 days (with a five day hiatus or "rest" interval between each cycle), using it with three ounces of gold chloride solution (in a concentration of one grain per ounce of distilled water) in the solution jar.

On *day one* of the cycle, I attached the copper electrode to the inside of my right wrist over the radial artery, which is the primary pulse point in the wrist (see Figure 1).

FIGURE 1:
ATTACHMENT OF THE COPPER ELECTRODE (WRIST).

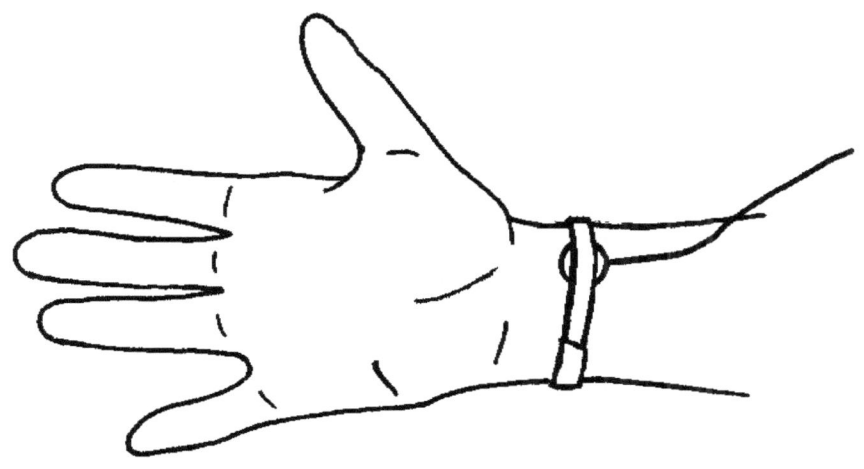

I applied the nickel electrode to my abdomen, slightly above and to the right of my navel (see Figure 2), putting a folded towel and pillow over it to keep it in place. Its application site was always the same for each day of the cycle (only the copper electrode changes position), and it represents the location of what the readings refer to as the "umbilical and lacteal duct plexus."

FIGURE 2:
ABDOMINAL PLACEMENT OF THE NICKEL ELECTRODE.

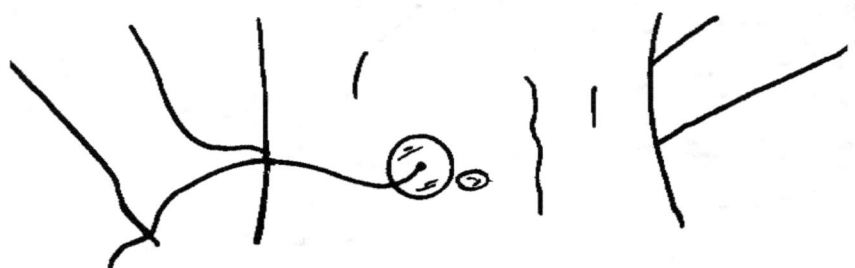

On *day two*, I attached the copper electrode over the radial artery in my left wrist.

On *day three*, I attached the copper electrode to the inside of my left ankle over the posterior tibial artery, which is the primary pulse point in the ankle (see Figure 3).

FIGURE 3:
ATTACHMENT OF THE COPPER ELECTRODE (ANKLE).

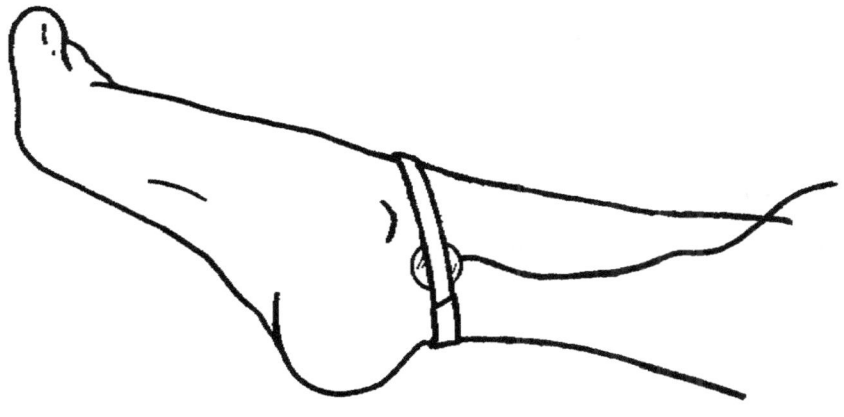

On *day four*, I attached the copper electrode to a comparable spot on my right ankle.

On *day five*, I placed the copper electrode on the inside of my right wrist again, and so on around each extremity for each day of the cycle.

At the end of the 28 day cycle, I would discontinue using the appliance for five days, after which I would repeat the cycle all over again.

TREATMENT RESULTS

I followed the above regimen faithfully, and within a few months I began to experience considerably less fatigue. Within two years, all signs and symptoms of multiple sclerosis gradually disappeared and have not returned – *except* for brief periods during and/or following certain viral infections (such as Herpes simplex), unusually stressful situations, when I do not keep up my treatments, or when I eat the wrong thing.

In my opinion, the basic cause of my condition has not as yet been corrected, just compensated for. Perhaps, as I continue to employ vibratory medicine, maintain good dietary habits, etc., the basic cause will be eliminated, and I will be "cured." In the meantime, I am quite content to be "just" in a state of remission, and if that state should continue indefinitely, I should be equally content.

Some individuals who have utilized the *wet cell battery* appear to have achieved a cure. Jess Belcher, for example (cited in Chapter 8), no longer uses the wet cell, and her symptoms have not returned.

O taste and see that the LORD is good: blessed is the man that trusteth in him.

Psalm 34:8

CHAPTER 8

OVERCOMING MS USING THE WET CELL BATTERY

The Meridian Institute (which is unrelated to Meridian Publications) was an organization in Va. Beach devoted primarily to researching the Cayce health readings.

In September of 1996, the Meridian Institute launched a *three phase* pilot study with nine participants to determine the efficacy of the Cayce treatment recommendations for MS.

The *first phase* consisted of a 10 day live-in period in which each participant received an initial evaluation of MS symptoms, an introduction to the basic Cayce diet, chiropractic spinal manipulation, abdominal castor oil packs, massage, colonic irrigations, daily sessions on the wet cell battery, and lectures on mental, physical, and spiritual aspects of healing.

The *second phase* consisted of a six month period in which participants were instructed to go home and adhere to the basic Cayce diet, make regular use of the wet cell followed by massage, attend to the mental and spiritual aspects of healing, and keep a daily log of treatments and treatment related events.

The *third phase* consisted of a three day live-in evaluation period.

Two participants did not complete the program, but, of the seven who did, *all* reported at least *some* improvement, and *three* reported *major* improvement.

Since it usually takes many months – if not years – to achieve the maximum potential of the Cayce method, these are impressive results! For a detailed report, see http://www.meridianinstitute.com/msreport.htm.

PHIL THOMAS' WET CELL THERAPY CENTER

Phil Thomas makes and sells the long-pole version of the wet cell battery (which he believes is superior to the short-pole version).

In 1993, he opened a wet cell therapy center in Virginia Beach for persons desiring to use the device.

He claims that a number of MS sufferers who came to the center experienced beneficial results.

One case in particular was that of Jess Belcher, who was diagnosed with MS at the age of 35.

Her symptoms included aching sensations in her legs, numbness on the left side of her body, losing her balance and falling, muscle spasms, headaches, and constant fatigue.

In addition to prayer, meditation, and dietary measures, she used the wet cell battery consistently for nine months.

She is now symptom-free and feeling fine.[1]

Another case was that of Maybritt Hansen, who was diagnosed with MS at the age of 37.

Her symptoms included tingling sensations, numbness, blurred and double vision, slurred speech, muscle weakness, poor coordination, loss of balance, mental difficulties, severe fatigue, foot pain, hypertension, paralysis, and bladder dysfunction.

In addition to herbs, flower essences, gem elixirs, amino acids and other food supplements, she used the wet cell battery for four months, alternating between the use of gold chloride, silver nitrate, and spirits of camphor in the solution jar (see http://tinyurl.com/hansen-ms).

---

[1] Deborah Seymour Taylor, "The Wet Cell Appliance," *Venture Inward*, July/August, 1993

In just a matter of weeks, she reported her progress as "phenomenal." [2]

Still another case was that of Astrid Scammell, whose symptoms included poor coordination, numbness, and foot pain.

After using the wet cell battery for a period of time, she reported a *marked* improvement in her condition. Even her digestion improved![3]

Phil Thomas' phone number is listed in the Appendix.

OTHER WET CELL SUCCESS STORIES

Down through the years, *many* persons afflicted with multiple sclerosis have been helped with the wet cell battery, either working independently, under the care of a sympathetic healthcare professional. or under the auspices of such organizations as the A.R.E. Clinic in Phoenix, or the Scottsdale Holistic Medical Group in Scottsdale, Arizona.

---

[2] Maybritt Hansen, "The Wet Cell: Overcoming MS," *Venture Inward*, July/August, 1993.
[3] Deborah Seymour Taylor, "The Wet Cell Rediscovered," *Venture Inward*, May/June, 1994.

CHAPTER 9

QUESTIONS AND ANSWERS
REGARDING
THE APPLIANCES

1 (Q) Are the radial appliance and wet cell battery officially "approved" medical devices?

(A) No; I am sorry to say that they are not. To properly evaluate them would require very costly long-term, large-scale, controlled studies which, so far, no interested party has been financially equipped to undertake.

2 (Q) Which version of the wet cell battery should I use, the long-pole or the short-pole?

(A) While the readings on MS do not specify which model is preferable, I am currently of the opinion that, though both devices may be equivalent from a purely *electrical* standpoint, the long-pole version may be superior from a *subtle energies* standpoint.

3 (Q) What is the purchase price of each appliance?

(A) As of this writing, the average price of the radial appliance and the *short-pole* version of the wet cell battery is under $240. The *long-pole* version of the wet cell is proportionately more expensive.

4 (Q) Can improper use of either appliance be harmful?

(A) Definitely. As anyone in the healing arts can tell you – and the readings stress this fact, too – any therapeutic modality that has the potential for *good* also has the potential for *ill* if misapplied.

5 (Q) Why is the radial appliance often referred to as the radio-active appliance?

(A) When used *without* the solution jar, it acts to *attune* the body – somewhat like tuning a radio to the proper frequency.

6 (Q) Suppose I fall asleep while attached to the device and wake up an hour or two later?

(A) To prevent such occurrences, it is a good idea to purchase and utilize a timer.

7 (Q) Can I share the radial appliance with someone else?

(A) No. The readings specifically advised *against* that practice because, once you use the radial appliance, it becomes part of you – as personal an item as your toothbrush.

8 (Q) Can I share the wet cell battery with someone else?

(A) It is apparently permissible in most instances, but I advise against it until more is known about this particular issue.

9 (Q) Is attitude important in using the appliances?

(A) Very much so, particularly when using the radial appliance. If a person maintains a positive, hopeful, expectant attitude, keeping an open mind to real possibilities, and praying to God for healing and restoration, the appliances are likely to be much more effective than if one is filled with doubts, fear, and unbelief. Negative thoughts – as well as negative emotions like anger and resentment – seem to build a resistance that is difficult (if not impossible) for the appliances to overcome. Some readings on multiple sclerosis stated that *nothing* could be accomplished until and unless negativity – toward situations, circumstances, self, others, and God – was dealt with and eliminated.

10 (Q) What if I accidentally *drop* the radial appliance?

(A) I have dropped my unit several times on the bedroom rug and in the yard (although never on a really *hard* surface), and, as far as I could tell, it did not seem to harm the device. Of course, if one or both terminals become damaged, the appliance will need repair or replacement.

11 (Q) Is there any way to "prove" that the radial appliance is working?

(A) Yes. The readings state that if the appliance is connected to an amputee, he or she will experience the presence of the lost limb. As far as I know, this test has never been performed.

12 (Q) Can I *recycle* the ice used with the radial appliance?

(A) Try to use a fresh batch each day. Small ice cubes are preferable to large ones, and *crushed* ice is better still.

13 (Q) Suppose the radial appliance does not receive any sun between treatments due to inclement weather or other causes?

(A) Use it anyway. Do *not* defer any treatments on that account. The same rule also applies if the wiring, electrodes, and loop of the wet cell battery do not receive any sun between treatments.

14 (Q) Should I discontinue using the device if I contract a cold, the flu, or some other infectious disease?

(A) If you are using gold chloride in the solution jar, the answer is "no." The readings suggest that administering gold vibratorially will help combat such infections. Once, for example, I developed a urinary tract infection. The bacteria causing it spread throughout my whole body and I developed septicemia. My temperature climbed at times to 103° F. To treat it, I used the radial appliance in the manner described in Chapter 7, ate light, nourishing meals (including quantities of lettuce), drank plenty of fluids (I found pineapple juice to be especially refreshing), took increased amounts of vitamin "C" and Atomidine, tried daily to work up a good sweat by walking (followed by a warm shower), gave myself an enema once a day after a bowel movement, took an occasional baby aspirin and employed an electric fan (to control my temperature), drank a cup of Saffron tea at bedtime, and – of no less importance – prayed for my recovery. Within ten days, I was completely well. While an antibiotic (most likely a sulfonamide) could have been enlisted to treat this infection, I feared the potential adverse effects.

15 (Q) If vibratory medicine can be used to treat systemic infections, could it be used to treat AIDS?

(A) I would not be at all surprised if it were successful in at least *extending* and making *more bearable* the lives of those afflicted with the Human Immunodeficiency Virus. As suggested by the answer to the preceding question, however, vibratory medicine usually is most effectively utilized in conjunction with other therapies.

16 (Q) Is there any alternative to using the *lead* loop in the solution jar?

(A) Yes. Nickel and copper loops may also be used. They cost more, but last longer. Lead loops are preferable, however, because they present a larger surface area to the solution in the jar, are perhaps less chemically reactive to it, and were the type most frequently recommended by the readings. (I have found nickel loops to be the most *practical*, however, and have used them almost exclusively.)

17 (Q) Why is it necessary to *sand* the electrodes and the loop both before and after use?

(A) To insure that the device is functioning at top efficiency. You only want *bright metal* next to your skin and in the solution jar.

18 (Q) Should I sand the electrodes, the loop, and (if applicable) the poles even through brand new and unused?

(A) Absolutely. Just because these items are brand new does not guarantee that they are bright and shiny and clean.

19 (Q) How do I keep my *fingerprints* from getting on the electrodes and on the loop, where they do not belong?

(A) When you sand these items, I *strongly* suggest you wear a pair of non-sterile, vinyl gloves (available at most pharmacies);

20 (Q) How do I repair an electrode when I have sanded off the head of the pin to which the wire is attached?

(A) Take the electrode to the hardware store and locate a 3/8" long, round head bolt (stainless steel for the nickel electrode and copper for the copper electrode) whose diameter is small enough to fit through the hole in the electrode vacated by the spent pin. Buy several bolts, because you will eventually need them. You will also need to buy two matching washers and a matching nut. Push the bolt through the hole in the electrode so that the head faces inward (that is, toward the body if it were in use). Put the two washers on the other end of the bolt and screw on the nut. Wrap about 3/8" of bare electrode wire around the bolt between the two washers. Tighten the nut, and you are back in business.

21 (Q) Should I keep a written record of my attachments to the device?

(A) Yes; unless you do, there will eventually come a time when you cannot determine where to place the copper electrode, because you *forgot* where it was the day before.

22 (Q) Should I keep a written record of my use of the compound in the solution jar?

(A) Yes; that way, you will always know when to change it.

23 (Q) What if I attach myself to the device and then realize that I have incorrectly positioned the copper electrode?

(A) Simply remove the nickel electrode from the body, correctly reposition the copper electrode, and then reapply the nickel electrode.

24 (Q) Suppose, in my use of the radial appliance, I accidentally apply the *nickel* electrode first?

(A) Unlike the wet cell battery, the direction of energy flow when using the radial appliance depends on which electrode is *first* attached to the body. Applying the nickel electrode first will, as it were, throw the appliance into "reverse gear," causing energy to flow from the copper electrode, through the body, toward the nickel electrode. This is the *exact opposite* of what you want, and is of little or no therapeutic value. Skip the session for that day, and continue in the correct manner on the following day.

25 (Q) What if, *after* my session on the device, I realize that the copper electrode was incorrectly positioned?

(A) Just forget about it and try in your next session to proceed in the proper manner.

26 (Q) Suppose, as I am preparing to use the device, the electrodes accidentally *touch* each other?

(A) You have short-circuited the device. Skip the session for that day.

27 (Q) If I get the "urge" to reposition the nickel electrode slightly, is it permissible to do so?

(A) Yes; it is probably your body's way of telling you that it *needs* repositioning. The placement shown on page 49 is approximately correct for most individuals, but the *optimal* placement varies a little from person to person.

28 (Q) When is the best time of day to implement my vibratory medicine session?

(A) In the evening before retiring. If that is not feasible, try at least to schedule it for the *same* time every day (I have mine in the morning after breakfast; it helps me through the day).

29 (Q) Will I feel anything while attached to either appliance?

(A) Probably nothing definitive, except for an occasional feeling of nausea (in which case see below) or an occasional slight tingling sensation.

30 (Q) Will it ever be advisable to *cut short* my session on the device?

(A) Possibly. The thirty minute time limit specified in this publication is a good safe duration for most people to use most of the time. However, there may be occasions when your body is, for one reason or another, unprepared for a full session, and will so indicate by either an *increased pulse rate or a feeling of nausea.* Just discontinue that session and resume your regular treatment schedule on the following day. If it keeps recurring, however, you may need to shorten the scheduled duration of your daily sessions and gradually work up to the thirty minute mark.

CHAPTER 10

MISCELLANEOUS
QUESTIONS AND ANSWERS

1 (Q) What about acupuncture, hyperbaric oxygen, bee venom, and other alternative therapies?

(A) Due to its complex, multifacted nature, MS may be helped by almost anything that stimulates the body's natural recuperative powers, that fosters physiological balance, that removes toxins, that improves circulation, that unimpedes nerve flow, and, in particular, that promotes good digestion and assimilation (because, in most cases, MS is basically a nutritional problem). Are these measured sufficient, by themselves, to overcome the condition? The readings would say "no." For, in response to questions about other approaches to treating MS, the readings indicated that they did not supply "that needed" to permit the continual process of myelin renewal, hence its degeneration and removal by immune system cells.

2 (Q) What about Avonex, Betaseron, and other "Disease Modifying Drugs"?

(A) In my opinion, these medications do not accomplish anything that cannot be accomplished by other, more natural means – at far less expense and with far fewer (if any) adverse effects.

3 (Q) What do the readings say about smoking?

(A) The readings say that smoking in *moderation* (three or four cigarettes a day) is not harmful. However, they were referring to cigarettes devoid of additives or fillers, which are very difficult to obtain today. Besides, how many smokers do so in moderation? Edgar Cayce (who was not always successful in following his own readings) certainly did not, and it definitely shortened *his* life. Smoking killed my poor mother who, in the last days of her life, had to *fight* for every breath. Don't let that happen to you. *Don't smoke!*

4 (Q) What about water quality in this country?

(A) It is apparently much worse than most people realize. The readings advised drinking *boiled* water. In my opinion, due to pesticide runoff and other factors, the safest water to drink now is *distilled* (available at most pharmacies and supermarkets). Not all brands are of consistent quality, however. If it makes you thirsty, leaves an unpleasant aftertaste, or causes other untoward reactions, try another brand.

5 (Q) Should I stay out of the sun?

(A) In general, the Cayce readings advise avoiding direct sunlight between mid-morning and mid-afternoon. Depending on the season of the year and the latitude of your locale, however, you might want to avoid direct exposure to the sun except during the early morning and late afternoon (unless you are wearing sunscreen and/or protective clothing). Sunlight is good for you, and you need it to be healthy. Just be careful *when* you get it!

6 (Q) Are there any exercises that would be helpful?
   (A) If you are physically able, *walking* (especially for a mile after dinner) is the *best* exercise (if need be, in a pattern of walk and rest, walk and rest); also good are *swimming*, and *stretching* (like a cat).

7 (Q) Do the readings give any advice about losing weight?
   (A) Yes. In addition to eating along the lines suggested in Chapter 4, half an hour before each meal and at bedtime, drink one ounce of water mixed with three ounces of grape juice (preferably Welch's). This simple concoction helps prevent the food you eat from being converted to fat. It might also be a good idea to supplement your diet with chromium on a daily basis. It appears to help normalize blood glucose (sugar) levels. Many have experienced healthful weight reduction by utilizing the radial appliance *without* the solution jar.

8 (Q) Can you suggest a good *cleansing* diet?
   (A) Yes. Eat nothing but raw, organic Delicious apples for three days (if they are not organic, peel them). During this period, drink nothing but water. On the evening of the third day, take two tablespoonsful of extra virgin olive oil. (If possible, obtain a colonic irrigation the next morning.) The readings claimed that this regimen would detoxify *any* system. It is probably wise

to go on this diet *before* instituting *any* of the treatment recommendations suggested in this publication, and then again two or three times a year.

9 (Q) What is celiac disease and how is it related to multiple sclerosis?

   (A) Celiac disease (also known as celiac sprue and gluten intolerance) is a disorder characterized by an intolerance to the *gluten* in all forms of wheat, rye, barley, oats, and related hybrid grains. Ingesting gluten causes an immune system response that *damages* the absorptive lining of the small intestine (abstaining from gluten is normally followed by regeneration of the lining). One major consequence of this damage is the *malabsorption of food*, leading to possible deficiencies in vitamins, minerals (including, I believe, gold), fatty acids, and other important nutrients. Depending on the deficiencies involved, a celiac may develop night blindness, depression, bleeding tendencies, osteoporosis, rickets (in children), insomnia, muscle spasms, numbness, tingling, chronic fatigue, muscle weakness, bone pain, failing memory, irregular heartbeat, and a host of other health problems (including, I believe, MS). Another major consequence of this intestinal damage is that it often causes *sensitivities to other foodstuffs*, such as dairy, soy, and citrus products, tomatoes, and sugar. In November of

1988, I discovered that I am not only gluten-intolerant, but that I also have a number of associated food sensitivities. Since modifying my diet to exclude gluten, dairy, soy, and other offending foods, I have experienced a noticeable improvement in my general health and well being. It is worth noting that there are some striking similarities between celiac disease and MS. For example, the tendency to develop both conditions is present at birth; the onset of both may be caused by childbirth, trauma, certain viral infections, and other major stressors; tissue damage in both involves the immune system; both often involve the liver, spleen, and pancreas; both may present similar symptoms; and the symptoms of both tend to be relieved by drugs that suppress the immune system. The prevalence of celiac disease in the U.S. is estimated to be about 1 in 250. In my opinion, future research will reveal a substantially greater prevalence among persons with MS, and that *celiac disease can and does produce nutritional deficiencies sufficient to induce the onset of MS in susceptible individuals.* I *strongly* recommend that *all* persons with MS be screened not only for celiac disease (which involves a simple blood test), but also for other food and substance allergies and sensitivities (any or all of which, at the very least, may be capable of exacerbating MS symptoms). For additional information about celiac disease and its connection with MS, read *Can a Gluten-Free Diet Help? How?* by Lloyd Rosenvold, M.D. (available from Amazon.com).

10 (Q) You mentioned meditating while on the appliance. What is it and how do I do it?

(A) Meditation is communing with the Divine within for health, strength, guidance, and healing. It is mentioned many times in both the readings *and* the Bible (the quote on page 10 refers, I believe, to this ancient practice). For best results, it should be practiced *daily*. For information on obtaining a *free* three audio cassette course, "Meditation Made Easy," write to the A.R.E. Search for God Program Office, 215 67th Street, Virginia Beach, VA 23451.

11 (Q) How is it that, at the age of 74, you look so young?

(A) I believe the way in which I use my appliance makes of it a "fountain of youth." The readings claim that a person can almost *double* his or her life span by the vibratory administration of gold and silver. I do not use silver with the device, but apparently gold by itself is able to keep me "young looking."

12 (Q) Apart from the radial appliance and wet cell battery, is there any other way to administer substances vibratorially?

(A) Yes and no. At the time the readings were given, there was a device produced commercially known as the "B" battery. It was used to help power the vacuum tubes in radio equipment. A number of readings (including one on MS) recommended it as a tool of vibratory medicine. It was very convenient to use because, unlike the radial appliance, it did not require the handling of ice and, unlike the wet cell battery, it did not require the mixing of chemicals. Unfortunately, it went out of production many years ago. Perhaps some enterprising company or individual will resurrect it, as plans and specifications for it must exist *somewhere*. Also, it is possible that one or more (or a combination) of the myriad batteries presently available would suffice as a vehicle for vibratory medicine – an intriguing question which, hopefully, will be addressed and resolved by future research.

13 (Q) Is there any tangible evidence to suggest that the *liver* is involved in many cases of multiple sclerosis?

(A) Yes. There tends to be a *hardening* of the ductal system associated with the gall bladder (predisposing the gall bladder to infection) and of that portion of the liver surrounding the hepatic duct.

14 (Q) What is the chief *drawback* of vibratory medicine?

(A) Its slowness, particularly in treating neurological problems like multiple sclerosis. It would seem that a number of individuals who received readings for MS became impatient, discouraged, and discontinued treatment prematurely. That is why the readings often advised *patience and persistence* in its application.

15 (Q) What are my chances of recovery if I employ vibratory medicine?

(A) Despite the present paucity of hard data on which to base a prognosis, my own personal feeling in the matter is that if you faithfully and conscientiously follow the treatment recommendations outlined in Chapter 4, your chances of experiencing at least *some* improvement in your condition – if not total recovery – are good to excellent. Bear in mind, however, that it may take *years* to *fully* reap the benefits of this endeavor.

16 (Q) Are there any *contraindications* to the use of vibratory medicine?

(A) Do *not* employ vibratory medicine if you
  (1) are pregnant,
  (2) are angry or upset,
  (3) have alcohol in your system, or
  (4) have just taken a dose of Atomidine.

17 (Q) What is Atomidine?

(A) An aqueous solution of iodine trichloride. When used full strength, it is effective as an antiseptic in treating minor cuts and abrasions. It can also be used in the solution jar of either appliance, and several readings recommended that it be alternated with gold chloride and/or other compounds in the treatment of multiple sclerosis. Greatly diluted, it can be taken by mouth to treat not only iodine deficiency states, but also (according to the readings) Ménière's disease, myasthenia gravis, various glandular problems, and a number of other conditions for which iodine has not as yet been recognized as being of therapeutic value. In several cases of MS, the readings recommended taking Atomidine by mouth, but *not* just prior to implementing vibratory medicine.

18 (Q) From a metaphysical point of view, why did I develop multiple sclerosis?

(A) It is almost certain that you need it for your soul development, and for that reason it is *imperative* that you include the mental and spiritual dimension in treating it. For example, read Exodus 19:5, Deuteronomy 30, and John 14-17, and *know* that the promises contained therein apply to *you*!

19 (Q) Where did the information in the readings come from?

(A) The source varied depending on the type of information being sought. In the case of the "physical" readings, Edgar Cayce visited "in spirit" the person for whom the reading was being given, performed a complete examination, determined the nature of the problem, ascertained the most appropriate treatment recommendations, and perhaps (as an aside) commented on the weather or soil conditions where the recipient of the reading happened to be living. When he awoke, he would have no recollection of this "visit," nor of anything said during the course of the reading.

20 (Q) How was Edgar Cayce able to perform this incredible feat?

(A) That is a question that can perhaps best be answered by the angel mentioned in Chapter 1.

21 (Q) What is your relationship to the Association for Research and Enlightenment?

(A) I am a Life Member of the A.R.E. and have been a student of the Cayce readings for over forty-five years. The information in the readings has helped me *greatly*, not only in terms of defeating multiple sclerosis, but in many lesser ways as well. In fact, it is safe to say that I owe my life to the readings.

22 (Q) Why do MS symptoms tend to worsen in relation to stress, certain viral infections and vaccinations against them?

(A) Some of the symptoms of multiple sclerosis (such as dry mouth, tremors, blurred vision, urinary retention, and constipation) are due to a relative *increase* in innervation from the *sympathetic* division of the autonomic nervous system (as innervation from the central nervous system becomes progressively less dominant). The effect of stress, certain viral infections and vaccinations against them is to cause a *further* increase in sympathetic innervation, thus potentiating these symptoms. Moreover, some viruses and their vaccines exert a direct or indirect *neurotoxic* effect. The combination of doubly increased sympathetic innervation *plus* neurotoxicity can aggravate (or cause to surface) a wide range of MS symptoms.

23 (Q) Why do antiviral drugs seem to help multiple sclerosis?

(A) By inhibiting viral infections, they tend to eliminate *that* source of increased sympathetic innervation and possible neurotoxicity.

24 (Q) Is there any *drugless* way to decrease heightened levels of sympathetic innervation and thereby reduce some symptoms associated with MS?

(A) Vibratory medicine represents a long-term solution to the problem. As a temporary palliative measure, you might try taking (as directed on the label) Passion Flower Fusion (available from the Heritage Store listed in the Appendix). It is a natural sympatholytic, relaxant, and anticonvulsant. The readings often recommended it in cases of epilepsy as a non-habit forming substitute for Dilantin and phenobarbital. It may also be helpful in curbing the muscle spasms associated with spinal cord injuries. As a non-alcoholic substitute, you might try Passion Flower capsules or tea (available at health food stores).

25 (Q) In treating MS, does the vibratory administration of gold have any effect other than tending to eliminate the lack of that mineral in the system?

(A) Yes. It also promotes *central nervous system regeneration*. For that reason, the readings very often suggested its use in treating neurological problems totally unrelated to gold deficiency states, such as Down's syndrome, polio, stroke, and spinal cord injuries.

26 (Q) Is it possible to *overdose* on gold administered vibratorially?

(A) Definitely. You may become headachy, develop a bad taste in your mouth, and experience other unpleasant reactions. To avoid that occurrence,
be sure to stay within the parameters of vibratory medicine specified in this book.

27 (Q) Do any readings on MS recommend taking gold chloride by mouth instead of (or in addition to) vibratorially?

(A) Yes, several. Apparently, in these cases, the gold
deficiency was diet-related, or at least could be
helped by an oral gold supplement.

28 (Q) Can you recommend a good laxative?

(A) Yes, Fletcher's Castoria (available from Amazon.com). I remember my mother giving this to me and my siblings when we were kids. Cayce was big on keeping up eliminations (as he called them). He also suggested drinking plenty of fluids, a diet high in fiber, salads with olive oil dressing, and, in stubborn cases, abdominal castor oil packs, enemas, and colonic irrigations. He maintained that an "internal bath" would be good for everyone occasionally, and warned that you should never go a day without at least one bowel movement.

29 (Q) If only the vibration of a substance (and not the actual substance itself) is transmitted into the body via vibratory medicine, how is it beneficial?

(A) My impression from the readings is that one or a combination of the following mechanisms may be at work in any given situation: (1) the body responds as if the necessary substance is physically present, (2) the body is stimulated to create the necessary substance, or (3) the body is encouraged to increase assimilation of the necessary substance. The readings indicate that, in treating MS with vibratory gold, the latter mechanism predominates.

30 (Q) Does *childbearing* put a woman at risk for developing MS?

(A) Yes. Depending on the circumstances, pregnancy can leave a woman *nutritionally bankrupt* and with certain glands that are *spent*. That occurrence, coupled with an MS predisposition, can trigger the condition. The prevalence of multiple sclerosis among young mothers just starting a family can be explained in this way. It also explains why women with MS experience a worsening of symptoms for *months* after childbirth.

31 (Q) Why do MS symptoms frequently abate during pregnancy?

(A) The glandular disturbance often associated with multiple sclerosis appears to be at least partially corrected or offset during such periods.

32 (Q) What is one of the best ways to *prevent* MS?

(A) Adhering to the dietary advice in Chapter 4.

33 (Q) What foods are high in gold?

(A) Shellfish, carrots, and salsify (oyster plant).

34 (Q) Why is MS more prevalent in some geographical regions?

(A) Some of the factors responsible may include variations in dietary habits, the presence of environmental toxins (especially mercury), genetic differences among groups of people, the lack of sunlight, and the ready availability of nutritionally deficient food (grown on depleted soil, milled, processed, and refined).

35 (Q) Why do women develop MS at a rate more than double that of men?

(A) I believe it is because women are more susceptible to glandular disturbances, are more prone to develop vertebral subluxations (due to greater joint laxity), and are more likely to be nutritionally compromised (due to relatively poorer diet, monthly iron loss, and the nutritional demands of pregnancy).

36 (Q) Why is muscle pain a symptom in some cases of multiple sclerosis?

(A) It may be related to the attempt on the part of muscle tissue to "wrest," so to speak, necessary nutrients from the surrounding circulation.

37 (Q) What is the relationship between vibratory medicine and energy medicine?

(A) Vibratory medicine is a *type* of energy medicine. The radial appliance and wet cell battery are basically energy medicine devices which, when used with the solution jar, become vibratory medicine devices.

38 (Q) Besides vibratory medicine, diet, and massage, do the readings consistently recommend any other therapy for MS?

(A) Osteopathic spinal manipulation was recommended in enough readings on multiple sclerosis (about 1 in 4) that you might consider obtaining (on a twice per week basis) a series of 6 to 8 general manipulations – including the sacrum and coccyx – *before* initiating your first vibratory medicine session, and two or three times a year thereafter. Unfortunately, very few osteopathic physicians currently practice spinal manipulation, so it may be difficult to find a suitable practitioner. (Some chiropractors and naturopaths are skilled in osteopathic techniques.)

39 (Q) What if vibratory medicine does not work for me?

(A) It is known that some individuals do not respond to vibratory medicine. Even so, if there has been absolutely no improvement in your condition after the first several months of treatment (assuming you were following all procedures correctly, your device was functioning properly, and all connections were good), consider making the following changes in the treatment plan:

(1) if you were using the radial appliance, try the wet cell battery;

(2) if you were using the short-pole version of the wet cell, try the long-pole version;

(3) if you were using the general approach to electrode placement, try the specific approach;

(4) if you were following Plan "A," try Plan "B;"

(5) if you were following Plan "B," try Plan "C;"

(6) increase the dosage of Atomidine to two drops;

(7) if you have not already done so, obtain the osteopathic spinal manipulations mentioned in the answer to the preceding question;

(8) strive to rid yourself of anger, resentment, bitterness, unforgiveness, prejudice, hatred, animosity, jealousy, hostility, unbelief in the efficacy of vibratory medicine, and all other negative attitudes and emotions;

(9) other options include increasing the duration of your vibratory medicine sessions, increasing both the size of the solution jar and the amount of solution, increasing the concentration of the solution, and alternating gold chloride with commercial strength spirits of camphor and/or a solution of silver nitrate (see the readings on MS for examples of these and other possibilities); and

(10) *above all*, get right with God by sending for, listening to, and heeding the counsel contained on the "Unshackled!" cassette mentioned on page 118.

40 (Q) Do you have any additional helpful advice?

(A) Yes. If you have not already done so, call the Multiple Sclerosis Foundation (1-800-441-7055), the Multiple Sclerosis Association of America (1-800-532-7667), and the National Multiple Sclerosis Society (1-800-344-4867) to obtain information regarding the many useful publications and services available from these organizations to persons with MS. Also, get plenty of sleep, and avoid stress, heat, viral infections, and overexertion. In addition, you might consider elevating the head of your bed 6" to 8" and wearing a copper bracelet (for MS-related inflammation), and supplementing your diet with the following (all of which are obtainable from the Heritage Store or other health food outlets): borage, black currant, or evening primrose oil (for omega 6 fatty acids), fish oil (for omega 3 fatty acids), colloidal gold, bee pollen (one of nature's most perfect foods), co-enzyme Q10 (the energy catalyst), alfalfa (a natural multivitamin/mineral), sunflower seeds (loaded with nutrition), acidophilus (a source of friendly intestinal bacteria), phosphatidylserine (said to be a brain food), St. John's Wort (for depression), Ginkgo Biloba (for mental difficulties), Milk Thistle (for liver health), Ginseng (for vitality), lecithin (believed to help nourish the nervous system), Jerusalem Artichoke (for pancreatic insufficiency), and Kava Kava, Valerian, and/or Chamomile (for insomnia). A wealth of additional information on the drugless management of MS may be found in Judy Graham's book, *Multiple Sclerosis* (available from Amazon.com).

41 (Q) How would you summarize the treatment recommendations presented in this book?

(A) First, go on the apple cleansing diet described on pages 70-71. Upon completion of the apple diet, implement the dietary suggestions on pages 32-34; at the same time, commence receiving the osteopathic spinal manipulations recommended on pages 82-83. When the first series of manipulations has been completed, begin using the wet cell followed by massage as suggested on pages 29-31. Two or three times a year, repeat both the apple diet and the manipulations. Eliminate *all* negative attitudes and emotions. Lastly – and most importantly – *make knowing God your highest aim.*

42 (Q) What do you forsee as the future of vibratory medicine?

(A) I believe that it will eventually be hailed as one of the greatest contributions to modern medicine since the advent of penicillin.

AFTERWORD

I have shared my successful conquest of MS with numerous MS sufferers (some of whom occupied wheelchairs and were in *pitiful* shape). Often, what I said seemed to go in one ear and out the other – as if they were destined *not* to overcome their condition.

Be the exception to the rule!

Do not be deterred by apathy, inertia, indifference, or the protracted nature of the Cayce approach to overcoming multiple sclerosis. For, in my opinion, in the present state of our knowledge, *there is no better alternative to treat the CAUSE of the condition.*

Therefore, do not delay!

The time to begin is now!

It is much easier for vibratory medicine to *halt* the progress of MS than – after the damage has been done – to *reverse* it. So, even if you cannot follow *all* the suggestions outlined in this book (such as receiving massage therapy after each vibratory medicine session), implement as much of the program as possible. Partial compliance with the Cayce regimen is far better than total non-compliance. You *owe* it to yourself *and* to your loved ones.

Vibratory medicine may not work in every case, but it works often enough that it should at least be *tried* in every case – and that includes *yours.*

And, as you patiently, persistently, consistently, and prayerfully make application of the suggestions in this book, *may God grant you the grace to be healed!*

APPENDIX

SOURCES OF INFORMATION AND SUPPLY

The radial appliance and wet cell battery (and their various solutions, chemicals, and accessories) are presently available from a number of suppliers, including:

(1) The Heritage Store (1-800-862-2923),
(2) The A.R.E. Bookstore (1-800-333-4499),
(3) Baar Products (1-800-269-2502),
(4) Phil Thomas (1-407-831-2896), and
(5) Tom Hildebrand (1-919-742-3379).

In general, due to the relatively unproven nature and value of the appliances, none of the above parties make any medical claims regarding them.

Additional information about the appliances may be obtained from the above sources, as well as from the A.R.E. Library (757-428-3588, ext. 7141), and the A.R.E. Circulating Files Department (1-800-333-4499).

Other items mentioned in this publication (such as Atomidine) may be obtained from the Heritage Store and the A.R.E. Bookstore. Many Cayce-related items are now also available from Amazon.com.

To obtain a wide variety of food supplements at fair prices, call Swanson Vitamins at 1-800-437-4148. You can also visit http://www.swansonvitamins.com.

BIBLIOGRAPHY

Baar, B., *Compilation of Readings on Multiple Sclerosis*, Downington: Baar Products, Inc.

Baar, B., *The Radiac Book*, Downington: Baar Products, Inc.

Bjork, R.O., *Multiple Sclerosis And How I Live With It*, Phoenix: Birchbark Press, 1978

Cayce, E.E., *Two Electrical Appliances Described in the Edgar Cayce Readings*, Virginia Beach: The A.R.E. Press, 1993

De Vries, J., *Multiple Sclerosis*, Edinburgh: Mainstream Publishing Company, 1992

Delany, D., "Glutamate Gloom," *Healthways*, June, 1976

Delany, D., "New Hope for Headache Sufferers," *Health World*, Winter, 1986/87

Delany, D., "The Ultimate Fulfillment," *Venture Inward*, September/October, 1988

Delany, D., "An Alternative Therapy: Vibratory Gold," *Virginia Nurses Today*, July/August/September, 1997

DeMarco, T., "Favorable Results in Field Test of the Impedance Device," *Venture Inward*, May/June, 1989

Frankel, D., *Living with MS*, New York: The National Multiple Sclerosis Society, 1994

Gabbay, S., *Nourishing the Body Temple*, Virginia Beach: The A.R.E. Press, 1999

Grady, H., "The Cayce Impedance Device: A Gift on the Doorstep," *Venture Inward*, May/June, 1989

Graham, J., *Multiple Sclerosis*, Rochester: Healing Arts Press, 1989

Iams, B.A., *From MS to Wellness*, San Diego: Iams House, 1997

Karp, R.A., *Edgar Cayce Encyclopedia of Healing*, New York: Warner Books, 1986

Lieberman, S., and Bruning, N., *The Real Vitamin and Mineral Book*, 2nd Edition, Garden City Park: Avery Publishing Group, 1997

Mabery, M.V., *Inner Cycles of Health: Living with Multiple Sclerosis*, Waldorf: 21st Century Online Publishing, 1996

McGarey, W.A., *Physician's Reference Notebook*, Virginia Beach: The A.R.E. Press, 1983

McMillin, D., and Richards, D.G., *The Radial Appliance and the Wet Cell Battery*, Virginia Beach: Lifeline Press, 1994

Pageler, J., *New Hope And Real Help For Those Who Have Multiple Sclerosis*, 4th Edition, Pinellas Park: John Pageler, 1996

Pahnke, W.N., *Multiple Sclerosis Research Bulletin*, Virginia Beach: The Edgar Cayce Foundation, 1990

Parisen, B., and B., "Our Experiences with the Radio-Active Appliance," *The A.R.E. Journal*, March, 1978

Reilly, H.J., and Brod, R.H., *The Edgar Cayce Handbook for Health Through Drugless Therapy*, New York: Macmillan Pub. Co., 1975

Richards, D.G., "The Radio-Active Appliance Really Works," *Venture Inward*, March/April, 1996

Richards, D.G., McMillin, D.L., Mein, E.A., Nelson, C.D., *Research Report on Multiple Sclerosis*, Virginia Beach: Meridian Institute, 1997

Rosenvold, L., *Can a Gluten-Free Diet Help? How?*, New Caanan: Keats Publishing, 1992

Rowland, L.P., Editor, *Merritt's Textbook of Neurology*, 9th Edition, Philadelphia: Williams & Wilkins, 1995

Stearn, J., *Edgar Cayce – The Sleeping Prophet*, New York: Bantam Books, 1967

Sugrue, T., *The Story of Edgar Cayce – There is a River*, Virginia Beach: The A.R.E. Press, 1973

Thomas, R., *The Natural Way With Multiple Sclerosis*, Rockport: Element Books, 1995

Turner, G.D., and St. Clair, M.G., *Individual Reference File of Extracts from the Edgar Cayce Readings*, Virginia Beach: The Edgar Cayce Foundation, 1976

Wagner, K., "Alternative MS Treatment Works For Therapist," *Port Folio*, April 1, 1997

Wolfenden, A., "There *Is* Hope For MS," *Dimensions*, June, 1996

Copies of most of the *books* listed in this section may be purchased from either the Heritage Bookstore, the A.R.E. Bookstore, or Amazon.com.

Copies of most of the *articles* listed in this section may be purchased from the A.R.E. Library (757-428-3588, ext. 7141).

INDEX

A

R

ABOUT
THE
AUTHOR

Dr. Dudley Delany is a retired chiropractor, massage therapist, and registered nurse. He is also a born-again Christian whose testimony was broadcast world-wide in 1974 on the dramatic radio series, "Unshackled!" A 2011 graduate of the BBN Bible Institute and an ordained minister, he pastored the Hilltop Gospel Church of Virginia Beach until he retired in July of 2014.

The author *welcomes* your questions, comments, and suggestions. Please direct your correspondence to him via e-mail: dudleydelany@webtv.net

HELPFUL LINKS

http://tinyurl.com/about-ec

https://groups.yahoo.com/neo/groups/tecvl/info

http://tinyurl.com/ecs-ms-tx

http://www.meridianinstitute.com/msreport.htm

http://tinyurl.com/ecs-ms-tx-group

http://www.baar.com

http://www.happyhillspringworks.com

http://www.heritagestore.com

http://www.cayceconcepts.com

http://tinyurl.com/my-advice-to-msers

http://tinyurl.com/inflammatory-food

http://tinyurl.com/todays-modern-food

http://tinyurl.com/dump-gmos

http://www.mcmillinmedia.com/appliances

http://tinyurl.com/hansen-ms

For God so loved the world, that
he gave his only begotten Son, that
whosoever believeth in him should
not perish, but have everlasting
life.

John 3:16

NOTES